STOP SMOKING OR DIE!

HOW TO STOP SMOKING AND KILL THOSE NASTY CRAVINGS IN 30 MINUTES

JOHN GIANETTI

CONTENTS

Introduction	v
1. Proven To Work Method To Quit Smoking Naturally	1
2. A Quick Reminder Of What Cigarettes Are Doing To You	6
3. Overpowering The Withdrawal Period	8
4. The Modern Medical Strategies To End Cigarette Smoking	11
5. 10 Things You'll Notice Once You Quit Smoking	15
Afterword	23

INTRODUCTION

Regardless if you are a teen or a pack-a-day smoker, it can be very difficult to quit the habit. However, once you learn and acknowledge your options and prepare to quit, the process would be easier. As long as you have the right game plan that suits your needs, you can break free from your smoking addiction and manage your nicotine cravings like the millions of people who have already quit smoking for good.

Smoking cigarettes or tobacco is considered a psychological habit, as well as a physical addiction. Nicotine from cigarettes provides a smoker an addictive high, which is temporary. When you start getting rid of your regular intake of nicotine, it will cause physical withdrawal symptoms and cravings. Addiction to nicotine may come from the substance's "feel good" effect on your brain. When you smoke cigarettes, you feel that you can cope with depression, stress, boredom, or anxiety better.

Concurrently, you may have considered the act of smoking as part of your daily ritual. For instance, you may tend to smoke a cigarette automatically when drinking your morning coffee. You may also find it instantaneous to light up a cigarette while taking a break from work or school. Some people smoke cigarettes on their way home after a long day. In some cases, people smoke cigarettes as a way to relate or connect with friends, family members, or relatives who are also smokers.

In order to quit smoking successfully, it is necessary to address both your addiction and your routines that go along with the habit. In this book, "The Easy Way to Quit Smoking & Overpower Your Cravings FOREVER: Be Healthier, Live Longer, and Stop Smoking," you will be able to learn various information on cigarettes and the act of smoking through the following topics:

- The Best Ways To Quit Naturally
- A Reminder Of What Cigarettes Are Doing To You
- DO NOT Forget This When Quitting Smoking
- The Modern Medical Strategies To End Cigarette Smoking
- All Natural Methods to Help You Quit Smoking
- Lifestyles Strategies To Aid You When Quitting
- How To Save Yourself And Your Body Once You Quit Smoking

Follow these guidelines and you will stop smoking and kill those nasty cravings in 30 minutes!

1

PROVEN TO WORK METHOD TO QUIT SMOKING NATURALLY

Although some people have successfully kicked the habit of smoking through cold turkey, many smokers need to come up with a plan to keep themselves from lighting up a cigarette. There are various methods to quit smoking. These methods can be better implemented with a good plan that can address both the short-term and long-term challenges of smoking.

The top recommended methods to quit smoking successfully and naturally through a tailored plan specifically for your needs and smoking habits include the following:

1. **Ask yourself these questions about your smoking habit** – When you decide to quit smoking, you should be able to allot time for yourself to think of what kind of smoker you are; why do you smoke; and which events or moments of your life urge you to light up a cigarette. These questions will be able to aid you

in identifying the right techniques or therapies that are most beneficial for you. Some of the questions you should ask yourself include:

- Are you a social smoker?
- Do you feel the necessity to smoke before or after every meal?
- Do you have the urge for cigarettes when you are depressed, stressed, or anxious?
- Do you have an extreme addiction for smoking or a simple amount of nicotine will suffice?
- Are their specific places, people, or activities that you feel you should associate with smoking?
- Are you agreeable to acupuncture or hypnotherapy to quit smoking?
- Do you have other addictions such as gambling or alcohol that you associate with smoking?
- Are you interested in taking a fitness program?
- Are you open to talking about your smoking addiction with a counselor or therapist?

2. **Begin your plan with START** – Although you have already decided to quit smoking, doing it can be very difficult to do. As such, you need to begin with a START:

S – Set a date for quitting.

Two weeks from the day you decided to quit, choose a date to begin so that you still have enough time to prepare. Within these two weeks, you should not lose your motivation to quit. If you smoke at work most of the time, then set a date that falls on a weekend. This way, you still have a few days to adapt to the change.

T – Tell family, friends, and co-workers about your plan to quit smoking.

Allow your family and friends to get into your plan to kick the habit of smoking. Let them know that you need their encouragement and support. If possible, choose a quit buddy who also wants to stop smoking for good. This way, you can help each other go through the changes.

A – Anticipate and prepare for the changes and challenges you will encounter while quitting cigarettes.

It will do you so much help to quit smoking if you prepare for common changes and challenges ahead. Some of these include cigarette cravings, nicotine withdrawal, and restlessness among others.

R – Remove cigarettes along with other tobacco products from your home, work, car, or other areas you are always going to.

Discard all your cigarettes including your "emergency pack," matches, lighters, and ashtrays. You should also freshen up the areas that smell like smoke along with your clothes. Wash your clothes, shampoo your car, steam your furniture, and clean your carpet and drapes to eliminate smoke odor.

Talk to a health expert or doctor about helping you quit smoking.

Doctors and health experts can aid you to quit smoking by prescribing medication or suggesting other healthy alternatives. Although you can purchase alternative products over the counter from grocery stores and pharmacies, it is still best to consult a health expert who knows what the best solution is for you. Some of the alternative products you can purchase over the counter include nicotine patch, nicotine gum, and nicotine lozenges.

. . .

3. Determine the things that trigger or urge you to smoke – In order to help yourself quit smoking, you need to identify the things that urge you to smoke. You should also include activities, situations, people, and feelings. It would help you determine what triggers you to smoke by:

- Securing a craving journal that can help you identify your triggers and patterns. For instance, in a week or so until your quitting date, keep a list or log of your smoking patterns. Take note of the moments in a day when you crave to smoke. Indicate the time, intensity of craving in a scale of 1-10, the activity you were doing when you began to crave, who you were with, how you feel during the craving, and how you felt after smoking.

4. Determine if you smoke in order to temporarily get rid of overwhelming or unpleasant feelings - Some of the most common reasons why people smoke cigarettes include discarding feelings of depression, fear, anxiety, stress, and loneliness even if it is only temporary. For instance, if you have a long, tiring day and nobody is there to accompany you to unwind, it would seem that lighting up a cigarette relaxes you, making such stick of cigarette your only friend. Although this may comfort you or provide you a feeling of relief, you should keep in mind that there are other ways to do away with unpleasant feelings. Healthier and more efficient ways of discarding unpleasant feelings include using sensory relaxation methods, practicing breathing exercises, and exercising among others.

Most people who have already given up smoking have

found alternative ways to manage difficult or complex feelings without trying to light up a cigarette. You should remember that there will always be a time that you would encounter unpleasant or painful feelings even if you have already given up smoking. Thus, it is necessary to think of positive or healthier ways that you can do to deal with unpleasant feelings instead of reaching for a stick of cigarette.

How to Avoid Things that Trigger Smoking

Most people who smoke have a habit of lighting up a cigarette while drinking alcohol or after every meal. There are several methods you can do to avoid things or even people who can trigger you to smoke.

- Switch to non-alcoholic drinks
- Drink only in areas where smoking is prohibited
- Chew on a cocktail stick or straw
- Snack on chips or nuts
- Replace smoking after every meal with munching on a square of chocolate, eating a fruit or healthy dessert, or chewing a stick of gum
- Let your social circles who smoke know that you are quitting the habit
- Avoid staying with other smokers in a car or during coffee break
- Find non-smokers during office breaks

2

A QUICK REMINDER OF WHAT CIGARETTES ARE DOING TO YOU

Pipe tobaccos, cigars, and cigarettes are all made from dried tobacco leaves and other ingredients that give flavor. The smoking coming from these products is a mixture of chemicals that are produced through burning of tobacco along with its additives. Many people are unaware that the smoke from cigarettes, pipe tobaccos, and cigars is made up of more than 7, 000 chemicals. Unfortunately, 60 of these chemicals have been determined as carcinogens or those causing cancer. Other chemicals in tobacco products cause lung and heart illnesses that are likewise deadly as that of cancer. In fact, you might be familiar with some chemicals in tobacco smoke, as you would encounter them often. Some of these include:

1. Benzene – can be found in rubber cement
2. Acetone – can be found in nail polish remover
3. Cyanide – can be found in pest control products
4. Formaldehyde – can be found in embalming fluid
5. Methanol – can be found in rocket fuels
6. Ammonia – can be found in household cleansers

7. Acetic Acid – can be found in hair dye

8. Carbon Monoxide – can be found in car exhaust fumes

9. Lead – can be found in batteries

10. Arsenic – can be found in rat poison products

11. Cadmium – can be found in battery acid

12. Naphthalene – can be found in moth balls

13. Tar – can be found in materials for paving roads

14. Nicotine – can be found in insecticides

15. Butane – can be found in lighter fluids

16. Toluene – can be found in paint

17. Hexamine – can be found in barbeque lighter fluids

These are just some of the chemicals found in cigarette or tobacco smoke. In addition, tobacco smoke also contains poison gas such as nitrogen oxide. The addictive ingredient is nicotine, which is one of the harshest chemicals contained in tobacco smoke.

On the other hand, the tobacco leaves that are used in making cigarettes contain radioactive substances. The amount of these radioactive materials depends on the soil where plants grow, as well as the fertilizers used. However, this also means that the smoke has small amounts of radioactive material, which smokers inhale into their lungs. The radioactive material builds up and eventually becomes a huge dose in the lungs. Several studies claim that the build of radioactive materials in the lungs could be the cause of lung cancer and other respiratory diseases related with smoking.

3

OVERPOWERING THE WITHDRAWAL PERIOD

More often than not, people who stop smoking experience various physical symptoms as the body withdraws from regular nicotine intake. Withdrawal symptoms from nicotine usually begin as quickly as 30 minutes from the last cigarette. The symptoms peak about 2 to 3 days after stopping to smoke. These symptoms can last for several weeks and differ from one individual to another.

When trying to quit smoking, most people forget that it does not come easy. This is because of the various nicotine withdrawal symptoms that include insomnia, cigarette cravings, tremors, irritability, anxiety, increased coughing, difficulty concentrating, fatigue, constipation, headaches, upset stomach, increased appetite, depression, decreased heart rate, nervousness, anger, frustration, and headaches among others.

If you are trying to quit smoking, you should not forget that it can be very difficult due to nicotine withdrawal symptoms. Fortunately, these unpleasant withdrawal symptoms are just temporary. In a few weeks, toxins will be flushed out from the body and the symptoms would eventually lessen or get better.

In addition, there are many ways to cope with nicotine unpleasant symptoms. The ways of coping depend on the symptom. For instance, when you crave for cigarette, you can try distracting yourself, wait for the urge to pass, or take a brisk walk. Usually, craving for cigarette lasts during the first week although it can remain for a few months. Other symptoms and ways of coping include the following:

- If you are having symptoms of irritability or impatience, then take hot baths, exercise, avoid caffeine, or use relaxation techniques. This symptom can last for at least 2 to 4 weeks.
- If you are having symptoms of insomnia, use relaxation techniques, avoid caffeine after 6 o'clock in the evening, or read when it is difficult to sleep.
- If you are having symptoms of fatigue, then do not push yourself too much on work or other strenuous activities. Try taking naps. This symptom can last up to 4 weeks.
- If you are having symptoms of lack of concentration, then avoid stress or reduce workload. This symptom can last a few weeks.
- If you are having symptoms of hunger, then drink low-calorie drinks or water or eat low-calorie snacks.
- If you have coughs, nasal drip, or dry throat, then use cough drops or drink plenty of fluids.

- If you are having symptoms of constipation, then add fiber to your diet, exercise, or drink plenty of fluids.

4
THE MODERN MEDICAL STRATEGIES TO END CIGARETTE SMOKING

There are various methods that have been proven to be successful in helping people quit the habit of smoking. These include going on cold turkey; reducing intake of nicotine gradually in a short period; systematically decreasing the number of cigarettes smoked in a day; using nicotine replacement therapy or non-nicotine medications; and trying acupuncture, hypnosis, counseling through cognitive behavioral techniques.

Nowadays, there are different methods that you can employ to help you quit smoking. These methods can be modern medical methods or traditional all natural methods.

Some of the modern medical methods include medications such as nicotine replacement therapy, non-nicotine medication, behavioral therapy, and hypnosis.

- Nicotine replacement therapy – This modern method involves the replacement of cigarettes with substitutes such as nicotine patch or

nicotine gum. It delivers small and steady doses of nicotine to the body in order to relieve some withdrawal symptoms, less the poisonous gases and tars in cigarettes. This modern method helps smokers focus on dealing with psychological addiction. More so, this method can help smokers concentrate on new behaviors, as well as coping skills.
- Non-nicotine medication – This modern method helps smokers by reducing withdrawal symptoms and cigarette cravings without using nicotine. Some of the common medications of this method include varenicline (Chantix) and bupropion (Zyban), which are intended only for short-term use.
- Cognitive behavioral therapy – This modern method involves employing therapy for habitual behaviors associated with smoking. It focuses on breaking habits or learning new coping skills.
- Hypnosis – This modern method is one of the most popular options for those who want to stop smoking. It works deeply in a person's relaxed state. The individual is open to suggestions so the hypnotists can strengthen your determination to quit, as well as increase negative feelings toward cigarettes.

On the other hand, you can also opt for traditional or all natural methods to stop smoking. These methods include acupuncture, motivational therapies, cold turkey, and herbal supplements, and self-help books.

- Acupuncture – This all natural method is considered as one of the oldest medical techniques, which works by triggering the release of natural pain relievers or endorphins that allow your body to relax. It can help by managing smoking withdrawal symptoms.

- Motivational therapies – This traditional method involves self-help books that provide various ways to motivate you to stop smoking. One of the examples of motivational therapies is calculating monetary savings. You could be motivated to stop smoking by calculating how much money you could save without buying cigarettes.

- Cold turkey – This traditional method is probably the most common among people who have decided to quit smoking. It is driven by willpower. In fact, it has been determined that 85% of long-term quitters have gone cold turkey on cigarettes.

- Herbal supplements – This all-natural method is probably the healthiest alternative to anti-smoking medications or drugs. Some of the herbs you can use to aid you in quitting cigarettes include motherwort, valerian, and lobelia. These herbs have been found to fight anxiety, depression, and stress along with other common side effects of nicotine withdrawal.

5

10 THINGS YOU'LL NOTICE ONCE YOU QUIT SMOKING

Since you have already acknowledged that smoking is bad for the health, then you also acknowledge living a healthy lifestyle. Choosing to stop smoking is relevant to a healthier state of various aspects in life. Thus, when you stop smoking, your life would be so much better and healthier.

There are several aspects in your life that you can either choose to stay healthy once you quit smoking or make them worse when you continue to do so. These include the following:

- Sexual intercourse – When you stop to smoke, you improve the blood flow of your body. As such, it can also improve your sensitivity. More often than not, men who quit smoking get better erections while women find improvement in their orgasms and are aroused easily. Non-smokes are 3 times more appealing to prospective partners as compared to smokers.
- Improved skin condition – When you stop to

smoke, your facial ageing slows, as well as the appearance of wrinkles. Once you become a non-smoker, you can get more nutrients such as oxygen. In addition, quitting cigarettes can reverse lined complexion to smoother and younger-looking skin.

- Improved fertility – When you stop to smoke and decide to have a child, it can be easier to get pregnant as compared to smokers. Quitting cigarettes can improve the womb's lining, as well as allow the sperm of men to be more potent. It also increases the chances of conceiving through IVF and reduces the possibility of miscarriage. Moreover, quitting cigarettes can improve the chances of giving birth to a healthy child.
- Better respiratory condition – When you stop smoking, you can breathe more easily as the capacity of the lungs begin to improve by 10% within a span of 9 months. If you are in your 20s and 30s, the smoking effect on the capacity of your lung may not be noticeable given that you can still run or do tedious activities. However, lung capacity begins to diminish as you age. By the time that you are in your late 40s, your maximum lung capacity can have a huge difference between living an active, healthy life and having to wheeze while you go for a walk.
- Healthier, whiter teeth – When you stop to smoke, you lessen teeth stains and have a fresher breath. Non-smokers who used to smoke reduce the possibility of gum disease and teeth loss when they begin to quit.
- Reduces stress – When you stop to smoke, your

stress levels become lower. This is because nicotine addiction makes you stressed from the withdrawal of cigarettes. Since the levels of oxygen in your body begin to improve, you can concentrate better, as well as increase your mental and physical well being.

- Longer and healthier life – When you stop to smoke, you prolong your life. For instance, when you quit by the age of 30, you add 10 years to your life. When you are 60, you add 3 years to your life. As such, quitting the habit adds years to your life, as well as improve your chances of having a disease-free old age.
- Healthier people around you – When you stop to smoke, you not only make yourself healthier, but the people around you as well especially those close to you. Passive smoking can increase the risk of lung cancer, stroke, heart disease, and other illnesses in non-smokers. For instance, second-hand smoke can make children at risk of chest illnesses such as croup, bronchitis, and pneumonia. Children are also three times at risk of acquiring lung cancer in their later lives as compared to those who live with non-smokers.
- Improved senses of smell and taste – When you stop to smoke, you begin to boost your senses of smell and taste. This is because your body recovers from being dull due to the toxic chemicals in cigarettes.
- Improved and better energy – When you stop to smoke, your circulation begins to improve in 2 to 12 weeks. You may already notice that your physical activities such as walking and running

can be much easier. You also boost your immune system, which makes it easier to resist flu and colds. The oxygen increase in your body can make you more energetic and reduces chances of having headaches.

Chapter 6: 22 Ways To Save Yourself And Your Body Once You Quit Smoking

HERE IS a guide that you can utilize to gauge how long it would take to repair your body from the harm or damages that smoking has caused you.

1. In 20 minutes after quitting, you may notice your pulse rate, the temperature of your hands and feet, and blood pressure begin to return to normal.
2. In 8 hours after quitting, the remaining nicotine in your bloodstream drops by 6.25%; this is already a 93.75%-reduction.
3. In 12 hours after quitting, you may notice that your blood oxygen level increases to normal while your carbon monoxide levels drop to normal.
4. In 24 hours after quitting, you may notice that your anxieties would have increased its intensity; however, in about 2 weeks, it should return to near pre-cessation level.
5. In 24 hours after quitting, the damaged nerve endings would start to regrow while your senses of smell and taste go back to normal. You may

notice that your irritability and cessation anger, on the other hand, would have peaked.

6. In 72 hours after quitting, your body will be 100% nicotine-free as the nicotine metabolites would have passed through your urine. However, you may notice that the symptoms of withdrawal such as irritability, and restlessness pick up their intensity. You may also notice that your craving episodes would have peaked. Meanwhile, the lung bronchial tubes that lead to alveoli or air sacs start to relax as your withdraw from cigarettes. Your breathing would have become easier as your lung's ability to function start to increase.
7. In 5 to 8 days after quitting, you may notice having at least 3 episodes of cigarette craving per day. You might feel that minutes are like hours when in fact, a single craving episode only lasts for 3 minutes or shorter.
8. In 10 days after quitting, you may notice that your craving episodes reduce to 2 per day and occur in less than 3 minutes.
9. In 10 days to 2 weeks, you may notice that your nicotine addiction or craving episodes no longer occur. In addition, the blood circulation in your teeth and gums are comparable to that of non-smokers.
10. In 2 to 4 weeks, you may notice that your withdrawal symptoms including cessation anger, difficulty in concentrating, insomnia, depression, restlessness, anxiety, and impatience have already stopped. However, if by this period you still encounter any of these symptoms,

make sure to consult a health expert or physician.
11. In 21 days after quitting, brain acetylcholine receptor levels, which increased regulation due to the presence of nicotine, would have decreased its regulation while levels of receptor binding in the brains would have returned.
12. In 2 weeks to 3 months after quitting, the chances of heart attack have decreased and your lung begins to improve in functioning.
13. In 3 weeks to 3 months after quitting, your resistance to insulin would have gone back to normal even if you may have gained weight of about 2.6 kg.
14. In 8 weeks after quitting, your resistance to insulin would have normalized completely in spite of gaining weight of about 2.7 kg.
15. In 1 to 9 months after quitting, the withdrawal symptoms such as fatigue, shortness of breath, and sinus congestion would have decreased. Your lungs would have cilia regrown, which increases the ability of handling mucus. This would keep you lungs clean and resistant to infections. In addition, you may notice that the overall energy of your body has improved tremendously.
16. In 1 year after quitting, the chances of heart attack, stroke, and coronary heart disease would have decreased about half less than the chances of smokers.
17. In 5 years after quitting, the risk of subarachnoid hemorrhage would have declined to 59%. For women, the risk of developing diabetes is already comparable to a non-smoker.

18. In 5 to 15 years after quitting, the chances of stroke have decreased to that of non-smokers.
19. In 10 years after quitting, the chances of lung cancer have declined by as much as 50%. More so, the risks of mouth, throat, pancreas, and esophagus cancers would have declined, as well. The risk of developing diabetes is now comparable to that of people who have never smoked cigarettes in their lives.
20. In 13 years after quitting, the risk of losing teeth is comparable to those who never smoked as compared to smokers with 5.8 fewer teeth.
21. In 15 years after quitting, the chances of coronary heart disease are the same as those who have never smoked. The same goes with the risk of pancreatic cancer.
22. In 20 years after quitting, the risk of death in females due to lung cancer and disease would have reduced to the chances of those who have never smoked. The risk of pancreatic cancer would have decreased to that of a non-smoker.

AFTERWORD

Your body is smart enough to determine if it is being poisoned which is the reason why it could take time to get hooked on smoking cigarettes. When you first started the habit, your body might have encountered pain or your throat might have experienced burning sensations. In fact, you might have felt sick when you were starting the habit. This is just an initial indication that you should quit smoking. However, since you have chosen to continue, the body's alarm system has been turned off.

The consequences of getting addicted to smoking may be gradual. However, in the long run, smokers experience serious complications including stroke, heart disease, emphysema, and various cancers in the throat, stomach, bladder, and lung. In the same manner, smokers are always prone to infections including pneumonia and bronchitis. No organ in your body will be spared from the damaging effects of smoking. Just a stick of cigarette decreases your life span by 5 minutes depending on your manner of inhaling.

Now that your knowledge about smoking has been increased and the various methods of kicking the habit have been laid to you in the previous chapters of this book, it is time to reexamine yourself and take time to assess your ability to quit smoking smartly and intelligently.

You have already learned about the acronym START in Chapter 1 of this book. That is exactly what you need to do to help you quit. A quick summary of it is:

S – Set a date for quitting.

    T – Tell family, friends, and co-workers about your plan to quit smoking.

    A – Anticipate and prepare for the changes and challenges you will encounter while quitting cigarettes.

    R – Remove cigarettes from your home, car, and work.

    T – Talk to a health expert or doctor about helping you quit smoking.

These are the 5 important things that you should do to quit smoking smartly and intelligently. On the other hand, you also need to learn other ideas that may come hand in hand with these 5 important things.

For instance, your determination is a significant factor in order for you to quit smoking completely. To help you strengthen your determination, write down a goal statement of your firm commitment to discard cigarettes for life. You should have a goal statement that is similar to a dated entry in a diary. In your goal statement, it is advisable to express your feelings toward your desire to be a non-smoker. Write down positive feelings of accomplishing your goal, as well as how you feel now that you have discarded cigarettes from your life. You also have to state that you are looking forward to living the rest of your life with lighting up or even picking a stick of cigarette. Once you have written down your goal statement, keep a copy of it and read it as much as you want every day. It is best to read it when you get up in the morning and before going to bed.

Spend as much time as possible to affirming yourself repeatedly that you now have a new state of being; that is, being a non-smoker. Utilize daily affirmations for at least 4 weeks until you reach your quit date. This will allow your affirmations to reach your subconscious mind, which would eventually tell you that you are a non-smoker. Every affirmation you make would be instilled in your mind. After 4 weeks of affirmation, your thoughts would send out a new image of you as a non-smoker.

Through focused visualization, you can also reinforce a vision of yourself as not having to do anything with cigarettes at all. Create visualizations of yourself as a non-smoker. Try picturing yourself in different events and situations without holding a cigarette. For instance, picture yourself in a party, enjoying it, interacting with people without a cigarette, and going to bed with a smile on your face. Take time every day to visualize yourself as a non-smoker.

Finally, spend time to some effort to quit smoking every day. Make sure to reaffirm your drive to quit smoking. Picture yourself as a non-smoker and take time, even a few minutes, to repeat your goal statement and perform visualizations daily. Thus, the more effort you implement into kicking the habit of smoking, the greater your chances of success to be smoke-free for the rest of your life.

Remember to follow these guidelines and you will stop smoking and kill those nasty cravings in 30

www.ingramcontent.com/pod-product-compliance
Lightning Source LLC
Chambersburg PA
CBHW070037040426
42333CB00040B/1714